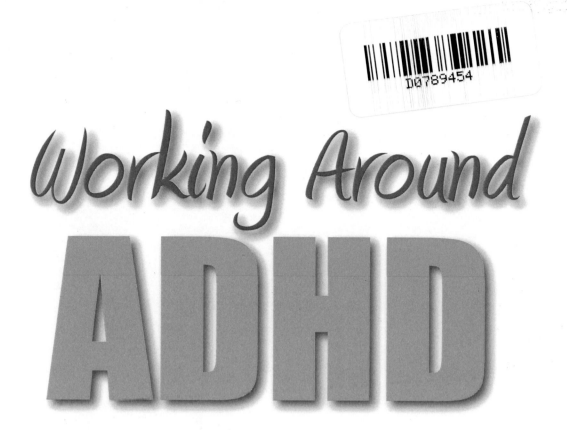

# Working Around ADHD

## How to take control, one obstacle at a time

# BILL ROLFE, PhD

Working Around ADHD: How to take control, one obstacle at a time.

Copyright © 2018 Bill Rolfe

All rights reserved.

Published by: Bill Rolfe
Los Angeles, CA
www.DrBillRolfe.com

ISBN: 978-0-9861863-0-1

Printed in the United States


Book Design: KarrieRoss.com
Images from istockphoto

For Moon

*I was trying to daydream but my mind kept wandering.*

*~Steven Wright*

# Is this book for you?

**Take The Test And Find Out**

Directions: Look at the list below. If you were to cross out any characteristics that don't really apply to you, how similar would your profile be to the one on the following page?

1. Able to pay for this book
2. Nonconformist, outlier
3. Good at estimating time
4. Sits still for long periods without fidgeting
5. Follows directions carefully
6. High tolerance for chaos & disorder
7. Spontaneous
8. Highly organized
9. Follows through consistently
10. Calm in a crisis
11. Attracted to shiny objects
12. Doesn't mind being bored
13. Inventive
14. Without looking, can list 3 crossed-out characteristics
15. Has ADHD (diagnosed or undiagnosed)

# This book is for you if you mostly resemble this profile:

1. Able to pay for this book
2. Nonconformist, outlier
3. ~~Good at estimating time~~
4. ~~Sits still for long periods without fidgeting~~
5. ~~Follows directions carefully~~
6. High tolerance for chaos & disorder
7. Spontaneous
8. ~~Highly organized~~
9. ~~Follows through consistently~~
10. Calm in a crisis
11. Attracted to shiny objects
12. ~~Doesn't mind being bored~~
13. Inventive
14. ~~Without looking, can list 3 crossed-out characteristics~~
15. Has ADHD (diagnosed or undiagnosed)

# Table of Contents

# Author's Note

I am a clinical psychologist, an educator, and now an author. I have ADHD, and this is my story.

I was 47 years old when I began to look into the possibility that I might have ADHD. I had been working in the field of psychology for twenty-five years. I was a baby boomer, a late bloomer, and I had earned my PhD in Clinical Psychology.

I was as confused as I was frustrated that my disorganization and chaos remained unabated despite professional training, personal therapy, and post-graduate schooling. It just didn't make sense to me how I, now Dr. Rolfe, was still losing my sunglasses, wallet, keys, and occasionally, my mind.

I spent a year just investigating ADHD. I read books, attended conferences, and I listened to audio recordings of lectures by the top leaders in the field. I listened to these recordings over and over and over again in my car. Finally, I began to *get it* what ADHD was. It also became clear to me that ADHD and I had a lot in common. My next move was to seek a formal diagnosis.

I was 48 years old when formally diagnosed with ADHD (inattentive type). I was relieved to finally have a name for what had been vexing me since childhood. The story of my life made so much more sense when I factored the influence of ADHD into the equation. Thus I began my *post-diagnostic honeymoon period*.

Alas, my post-diagnostic honeymoon faded with the realization that having the diagnosis of ADHD didn't stop me from losing my wallet, sunglasses, keys, etc. I still needed a treatment plan! I discovered, unfortunately, that most of the research on ADHD ignored adults altogether. *Adult* ADHD was still a novelty in the 90's. Essentially, adults with ADHD had only one viable treatment option, medications. I went to a psychiatrist specializing in ADHD who prescribed stimulants. I didn't think that the pills were working at first, as I didn't feel any buzz. However, I was accomplishing tasks rather effortlessly. Rather than buzzed, I was busy! I focused without straining, perhaps, for the first time in my life. This just seemed *too good to be true*, like I was getting away with murder. It took me a while to trust that stimulants were legitimate medicine, and that they were readily available to me.

Of course the stimulant honeymoon faded as well. Although stimulants can enhance focus they don't alter habits, expectations, or systems of organization. Since most of my habits had been deeply engrained long before I knew that I had ADHD, they were embedded with the false premise that I was a normal person!

I knew I would need to scrutinize all of my habits, beliefs, and systems of organization. I would have to find my own way forward.

One day I came across a most compelling research study by Paul Gerber and associates.[1] The study examined highly successful adults with ADHD and/or learning disabilities to determine if they shared any common factors. What they discovered was that these subjects **took control** by working around (and even exploiting) their "impairments" in order to achieve their goals. Researchers identified ten control factors linking these ADHD adults with successful outcomes. The control factors were processes or practices (EG: *recognizing, goal setting, and reframing*). These findings definitely caught my attention. I was especially intrigued by the idea of copying/adapting the ways of successful people with ADHD. Why not? These results were empowering, unconventional, and evidence-based. I was tired of always trying to re-invent the wheel. Here before me lay a set of wheels that had already been invented and proven Each control factor could be mastered by identifying and working around potential obstacles. My job was to engineer ADHD-friendly workarounds for each obstacle. I noticed that I felt that sense of control after successfully working around an obstacle. That sense of control went away, however, as soon as I tried working around more than one obstacle at a time. Taking on more than one obstacle at as time took me out of the present and bogged me down. However, I learned that I was able to remain anchored in the present even as I was progressing toward my future goal by only focusing on one obstacle at a time.

This has been a model that I have utilized both personally and professionally for many years now. I have seen many adults with ADHD take charge of their lives and work around their ADHD. Now you can do the same. This book is for you if you have ADHD and your wish to take control of your life. Each chapter represents a different control factor. Within the chapters are some obstacles and corresponding workarounds related to that particular factor. Now it is your turn to take control of your world by working around your ADHD. Just remember to focus on one obstacle at a time.

Bill Rolfe, PhD

[1](Gerber, 2001)

# Introduction

**Successful adults with ADHD took control of their worlds by working around ADHD employing these ten control factors[1]:**

Reframing ADHD

Recognizing ADHD

Accepting ADHD

Setting ADHD-friendly Goals

Managing Morale

Finding ADHD-friendly Pathways to Action

Finding Creative Solutions

Prioritizing Goodness of Fit

Cultivating Supportive Relationships

Practicing Persistence

As you work around the obstacles that arise within each control factor you will essentially be working around ADHD.

[1](Gerber, 2001)

# Utilize 10 evidence-based control factors to take control of your own world and work around your ADHD

The ten control factors from the research study have been assimilated into the structure of this book. Each factor is a chapter heading and is the theme for that chapter. Within each chapter you will find a series of ADHD related obstacles and corresponding workarounds associated with that particular factor. You can gain more control over both your internal and external worlds by working around the obstacles that relate to each factor. The key is to focus on one obstacle at a time.

# Experience taking control now!

> ## Who is the boss of you?

This exercise is designed to help you experience the subjective sense of agency that is related to taking control:

Imagine that you are driving to a very familiar destination in your car. The only caveat is that you have a passenger. Unfortunately, your passenger happens to be a whiny, obnoxious back seat driver who rudely demands that you turn left when you know very well that the destination is to the right. As you do it your way (turn right) the whiner says, "I told you to turn left and you turned right. **Who do you think you are?**"

Pause and breathe. Directing your attention to your body, say to yourself, *I am the boss of me.* Does this statement feel accurate? If you feel that *I am the boss of me* is an accurate statement then you are in a *taking control* state of mind. Notice the energy in your body. Now imagine yourself turning to the obnoxious, virtual, backseat driver and declaring with authority "*I am the boss of me.*"

Don't worry if you aren't feeling it. Try acting-as-if. Repeat *I am the boss of me*, a few times anyway. Imagine saying it to the whining backseat driver (even if you still aren't really feeling it). Notice the energy in your body as you act-as-if.

# Obstacle

**Focusing on your ADHD makes you feel out of control and helpless.**
Focused attention is a powerful force. Whatever you aim your attention at will tend to expand within your perception. When you focus intently on your limitations (ADHD) your sense of helplessness will expand. Western medicine may be re-enforcing your helplessness by defining ADHD in terms of the limitations it imposes on normal functioning. This outside-looking-in perspective is important for research and for making diagnoses, but not for empowering people with ADHD.

# Workaround

**Think of ADHD as just a series of obstacles to be worked around.**
This inside-looking-out perspective aims attention on possibilities instead of limitations. What expands is your sense of control. You don't have control over the limitations imposed by ADHD, but you do have control over generating possibilities (workarounds). Focus on those and you will feel in control and empowered.

*Think of ADHD as just a series of obstacles to be worked around.*

# Obstacle

**You get anxious and overwhelmed thinking about what lies ahead.**

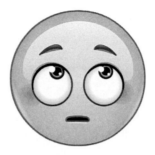

# Workaround

Your attention is residing in the anticipated future (where you have no control) versus the present (where you have control). Get into the present by focusing on workarounds, one obstacle at a time.

*Get into the present by focusing on workarounds, one obstacle at a time.*

# Obstacle

You have just been diagnosed with Attention Deficit Disorder
(ADD/ADHD). Now what?

# Workaround

**Pat yourself on the back for getting an official diagnosis.**
Now you can counter doubt with data.

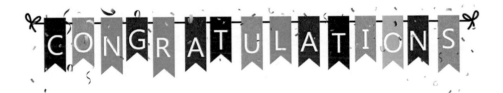

*Now you can counter doubt with data.*

# Obstacle

You believe that you have ADHD but you have never been formally diagnosed.

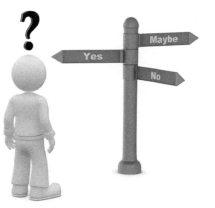

# Workaround

**Make an appointment with a health care professional who can diagnose you, then go in to get evaluated.**

The difference between having ADHD diagnosed vs. undiagnosed is comparable to the difference between marriage and cohabitation. Making it official makes a difference. It may be harder to summon the necessary resolve to work around ADHD if you don't know for sure that you have ADHD.

*It may be harder to summon the necessary resolve to work around ADHD if you don't know for sure that you have ADHD.*

# Obstacle

**There is no "cure" for your ADHD brain. Sounds hopeless.**

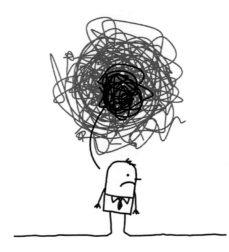

# Workaround

**This book will show you how to use your mind to work around the obstacles imposed by your ADHD brain.**

There may be no cure, but there are evidence-based strategies that enable you to take manual control over the neurological functions that are impaired by ADHD.

*This book will show you how to use your mind to work around your ADHD brain.*

# Obstacle

**You buy books but don't read them.**
You believe that you must always start a book at the beginning and read every word sequentially up to the last period.

# Workaround

**Go with the style of reading that is most natural for you.**
Different ways to read this book:
you could
    start at the beginning
      start at the end
        start anywhere
          read the chapter summaries only
            flip through the book until something catches your attention

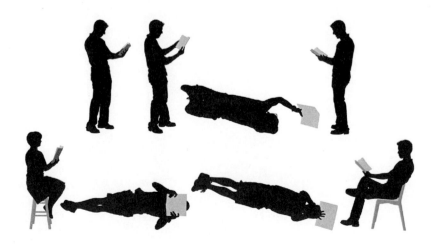

There is more than one way to ~~skin a cat~~ work around an obstacle.

# Chapter 1

# Reframing ADHD

A frame provides perspective for understanding something. Reframing involves changing perspectives. In this chapter (and throughout this book) we will be reframing ADHD as a series of obstacles to work around, ...one at a time.

This chapter will highlight workarounds for each of the following framing obstacles:

- ADHD ignorance abounds
- ADHD interferes with your perception of time
- Successes can lead to diagnosis doubts
- People interpret intention behind your inattention
- You harbor shame about having ADHD
- Your executive functioning is impaired by ADHD
- How you determine if a trait or behavior is an *ADHD thing*
- Why you should care whether or not something is an ADHD thing
- Unless you are using artistic license, don't blame it on your ADD
- Your mind will move toward chaos in the absence of external structure
- Your mind is susceptible to being organized by the environment you are occupying
- When normal people claim to have ADHD

# 1 Obstacle

**ADHD ignorance abounds.**
Even if you learn just a little about ADHD, you will probably know more about it than most people do. Most people (including health-care professionals) do not really understand what ADHD is. How much do you know about ADHD? By understanding what ADHD is, as well as what it isn't, you can begin working around it. ADHD is complex. There are those who will even argue that ADHD doesn't really exist. How will you determine if they are right or wrong unless you are informed yourself?

# Workaround

**Get informed (via your preferred style of learning).**
Keep reading this book.
Read other books.
Go to lectures.
Attend conferences (CHADD, ADDA).
Listen to podcasts.
Watch webinars.
Read blogs.
Talk with other people who have it.
Notice your own behavior patterns – keep a journal.
World Wide Web.
Stay Curious.

*Even if you learn just a little about ADHD,*
*you will probably know more about it*
*than most people do.*

# Obstacle

**ADHD interferes with your perception of time.**

People with ADHD are:

- Not so good at estimating how long it will take to get ready.
- Not so good at estimating how long a task will take to accomplish.
- Not so good at synchronizing *what to do* with *when to do it*.

# Workaround

**Train yourself (and others) to view any time estimations that you make with great suspicion.**

Externalize time. Learn to rely on time-keeping devices so that your mind is not burdened trying to keep track of time.

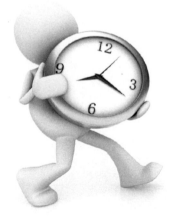

*Externalize time.*

# 1

# Obstacle

**Sometimes you doubt the validity of your ADHD diagnosis after achieving some success:**
"…If I am able to perform well I must not have ADHD."

# Workaround

**Think of ADHD as an *inconsistency disorder*.**
ADHD might be better understood as a disorder that is characterized by inconsistencies in performance more than by deficits in attention. Most of us with ADHD are able to rally and get it together to create order or to pay close attention if we are determined and the challenge involves elements of novelty or stimulation. Our ADHD is more likely to rear its ugly head, however, when we attempt to sustain that close attention over time (especially when the tasks are boring). Our problem is not about being able to perform. Our problem is about not being able to perform evenly.

### *Think of ADHD as an inconsistency disorder.*

# Obstacle

**People infer that there are sinister intentions behind your inattention.**

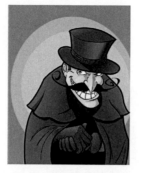

People (including psychotherapists) sometimes, out of ignorance, infer symbolic meaning behind your symptoms of ADHD. "You are self-sabotaging," or "You must have fear of success," or, "Your lateness is rude and tells me that don't respect my time," are examples.

# Workaround

**Protect yourself from toxic interpretations.**

Behaviors driven by restlessness, inattention, and/or impulsivity are devoid of any symbolic meaning. Could you imagine accusing the driver of a car with faulty brakes of *not wanting to stop*? Start by informing yourself about the nature of ADHD. Then your job is to become the gatekeeper (or bouncer) who carefully monitors, labels, and filters incoming communications. Toxic communications laced with judgment, guilt, or shame can be labeled and filtered out at the gate.

> *Behaviors driven by restlessness, inattention, and/or impulsivity are devoid of any symbolic meaning.*

# 1

# Obstacle

**You are ashamed about having ADHD.**
You feel defective.

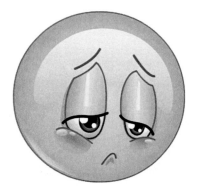

# Workaround

**Reframe your problem.  It is shame, not ADHD.**
You are not your ADHD. ADHD is something that you have, not something that you are. The only thing defective about you is your belief that you are defective. You can actually tame shame by labeling it in your mind. Identifying shame can also help you make sense of why you feel so bad, just as identifying dog doo on your shoes can help you make sense of why your feet smell so bad.

## *You are not your ADHD!*

# Executive Functioning

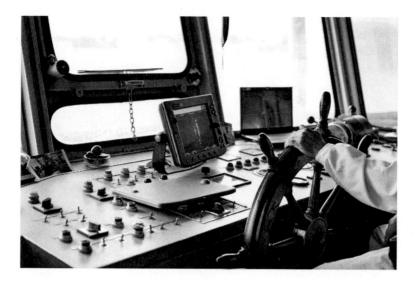

Imagine that you are the captain of a ship (a metaphorical way of understanding executive functioning). As captain you will be assuming your place at the helm, high up in the bridge. The bridge is where you have command of all of the ship's operations. The captain is especially active during transitions such as departures and arrivals. The captain predetermines the exact course to the destination, but is also prepared to work around unforeseen circumstances such as squalls, food poisoning, or pirates. The captain relies upon sophisticated electronics in order to guide the ship, unless he or she happens to have been assigned to the good ship *ADHD*. This happens to be the ship to which we were assigned. The good ship *ADHD* is seaworthy, but is equipped with unreliable navigational instruments. Nonetheless you, as captain, must work around the challenges imposed by faulty navigational equipment and bring the ship to port.

For humans the metaphorical bridge on the *good ship ADHD* is located in the region of our brain called the pre-frontal cortex. When you are the captain on the bridge this is the part of the brain you occupy. The sophisticated electronics, which automatically regulate your executive functions, have a glitch (ADHD). All of the areas affected are listed on the next page.

**1**

Here is a list of some

# Executive Functions

*Regulating emotion*
*Motivating self through boring tasks*
*Remembering the gist while engaging in the details*
*Estimating time accurately*
*Doing things in their proper order or sequence*
*Following through*
*Getting back on track despite interruptions*
*Planning*
*Organizing*
*Prioritizing*
*Self-monitoring*
*Getting started*
*Stopping*
*Transitioning*
*Delaying gratification*
*Pausing to think before acting*
*Following rules, or directions*
*Self-structuring*

# Obstacle

**ADHD impairs your executive functioning.**
Executive functions enable us to navigate. Inattention, restlessness, and/or impulsivity interfere with executive functioning. If you have ADHD, you have surely experienced executive function difficulties (see list on the previous page). Executive functioning is arguably the area most adversely affected by ADHD.

# Workaround

**Externalize executive functioning.**
The good news is that if you understand that your executive functioning is unreliable (when it is running on auto pilot) you can switch to manual control. You do this by mindfully directing your attention to the challenges related to planning, organizing, prioritizing, etc., and then experiment with some ADHD-friendly workarounds to manage those functions. Take control by externalizing as much as possible. You could, for example, externalize specific executive functions (like getting started, stopping or transitioning) by using timers. You could motivate yourself through boring tasks by breaking tasks into small chunks, or perhaps by putting on music or an old movie that you have seen many times. Find what works for you.

1

You are

OK

but

your

executive functioning

isn't

nonetheless

you do

remain

the executive

in charge

of

your

functioning

(and malfunctioning)

# Obstacle

**1**

**You can't tell when something is an *ADHD thing*.**
It can be a challenge to know whether to attribute a trait or behavior to ADHD or not. How can you tell?

# Workaround

**If the trait or behavior is related to an executive function, it is probably also impaired by ADHD.**
Look at the list of executive functions.

# 1 Obstacle

You don't know why you should care whether or not something is *an ADHD thing.*

# Workaround

**Linking a behavior pattern or trait to ADHD can help you:**
- **Make accurate sense of persistent patterns** "I was told that I have trouble finishing things because of *fear of success*. Now I know that I am tripped up by ADHD, not by some need to self sabotage."
- **Revise the your story of your life** "I had trouble focusing on schoolwork as a child because my brain was sluggish. I was told that I was being lazy, but now I know that I was actually trying very hard."

## Develop Workarounds

- **Adjust self-expectations** "I know that I won't remember those directions, so please write them down for me."
- **Build compensatory systems** "I run chronically late so, I will try leaving 15 minutes earlier than I think I should."
- **Have empathy for yourself** "No wonder I felt so misunderstood and ashamed. I was punished and criticized for something that I didn't have control over."
- **Be able to predict symptoms before they arise** "When I have *free time*, I tend to get very anxious and end up feeling paralyzed, instead of free. I know that this is related to being unstructured, so I am going to structure my *free time* ahead of time by making some plans with friends"

# Obstacle

**1**

Some people act as if ADHD gives them a pass on responsibility.

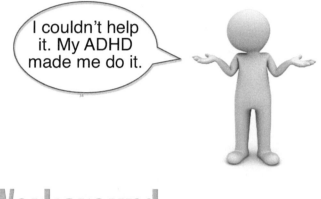

# Workaround

**ADHD is not an irresponsibility disorder.**
We are still accountable for all of our behaviors even though our ADHD symptoms are unintentional.

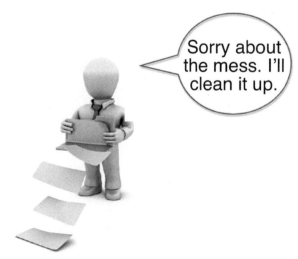

*ADHD is not an irresponsibility disorder.*

# 1 Obstacle

**ADHD minds tend to move toward *Chaos*
when disconnected from external structure.**

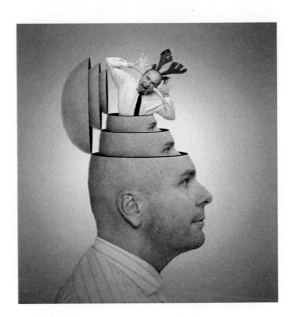

# Workaround

**Structure your *free time*.**
The idea of having some *free time* may sound attractive (especially when you are
thinking about it while in a structured environment).

*Free time* is likely to morph into *chaos time* unless you impose some structure.

## *Structure your free time.*

# Obstacle

**Your mind is susceptible to being organized by the environment that you are in.**

People with ADHD are usually able to sustain attention as long as the external environment provides the structure and reinforcement (EG: School or work can provide structure). It is only in the absence of external structure (when behaviors must be internally planned, organized, and sustained toward a future goal) that people with ADHD cannot perform consistently.

# Workaround

**Take control of your mind by choosing, or structuring, your environment mindfully. Place yourself in the environment that fosters the mindset you wish to have.**

EG: If you get more work done in a coffee shop or a library, then do your work at the coffee shop or library (the author is currently writing in a hotel room). You can also structure your environment just by putting on music in the background.

*Place yourself in the environment
that fosters the mindset you wish to have.*

# Workaround
## Experiment

**Structure your environment with music**

Instructions:

1. Find some music that can function as background music. Instrumental music is ideal, but vocals are also OK as long as they are not distracting. Make sure the beat matches the pace you want your mind work at.

2. Pick something (anything) around your home or workplace that needs to be repaired, cleaned, assembled, redistributed, or maintained.

3. Gather what you need in order to repair, clean, assemble, redistribute or maintain this thing.

4. Notice your mood, energy & motivation as you anticipate and actually begin.

5. Put on some kind of instrumental (non-vocal) music.

6. Pay attention to your mood, energy & motivation as you continue the same task, but with music on.

7. Some people with ADHD leave music on all day.

# Obstacle

**You don't know how to make sense of the fact that so many people casually claim that they too have ADD.**

# Workaround

**Having ADHD means that you are at the far end of a normal spectrum.**
You may hear people casually say, "I must have ADHD," when they lose track of something or are forgetful. Attention, like many things, resides on a normal spectrum. Being diagnosed with ADHD means that you are farther from the middle of the spectrum than almost everyone. Yes everyone has inattentive, restless, and/or impulsive moments. For people with ADHD, however, these moments are the rule rather than the exception. It can be very hard to fathom what it means to live with ADHD if you don't have it. People diagnosed with ADHD just have those moments much more frequently and far more pervasively than everyone else.

*Having ADHD means that you are at the far end of a normal spectrum.*

1

# Chapter 1 Summary
# Reframing ADHD

You need to know what ADHD is (and isn't) before you can work around it. Misinformation and ignorance abound about ADHD. I have even heard mental health professionals (my own brethren) declare, with authority, that ADHD is not real. It is because ADHD is a very complex disorder that **I believe that everyone who has ADHD is well served to become an expert on the subject**. Otherwise you may absorb some contaminated thinking. It is important that you have answers to misinformed comments like, "If it was important, you would do it," or, "If only you would apply yourself." It is also important that you understand yourself and make accurate sense of your life.

ADHD has nothing to do with intelligence, maturity, or intention. It is a performance disorder characterized by an impaired ability to internally organize and guide behaviors toward future goals. ADHD is also a chronic condition that is associated with behavioral inconsistency. The ADHD mind is vulnerable to becoming organized by the structure of the external environment that surrounds it. In the absence of external structure, the ADHD mind is likely to move toward chaos. You can use this to your advantage by choosing your environment based on the ways that it organizes your mind.

ADHD disrupts executive functioning. Understanding the relationship between executive functioning and ADHD can enable you to create effective compensatory workarounds. For example, you can use technology to help you with planning, prioritizing, timing, and remembering details.

Reframing ADHD can help you shrink rather than absorb shame. As you develop a deeper understanding of what ADHD is, you will be ready to take the next step, which is to recognize how when and where your ADHD shows up. You can't work around it unless you recognize it

# Chapter 2

# Recognizing ADHD

**Y**ou have to recognize ADHD before you can work around it. Recognizing involves mindful self-monitoring, a skill that can be learned and strengthened with practice. See if you can start noticing how, when, and where ADHD shows up in your life. Self-monitoring allows you to recognize and track its footprint.

This chapter will highlight workarounds for each of the following recognition obstacles:

- You are not familiar with ADHD's footprint
- You'd rather not know more about ADHD
- Monitoring ADHD when one of the symptoms of ADHD is poor self monitoring
- To work around ADHD you must pay attention to your mind
- You believe that you are not disciplined enough to start a meditation practice
- Impulsive, restless, and distractible people don't seem like the best candidates for meditation
- Judgment can be deeply engrained in you

# 2 | Obstacle

**You may not be used to tracking ADHD's footprint.**

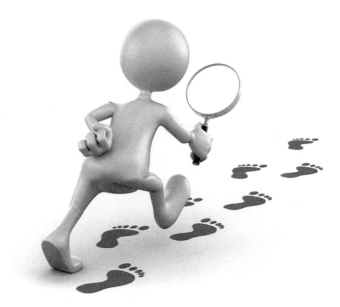

# Workaround

**You may begin to recognize ADHD's footprint simply by looking for it.** (If you set out to notice how many red cars are on the road you will start to notice red cars).

# Obstacle

Ignorance is bliss. You would rather not know how your ADHD is affecting you.

# Workaround

**Recognition can lead to greater self-control.**
Would you want to know if your vision was impaired ?

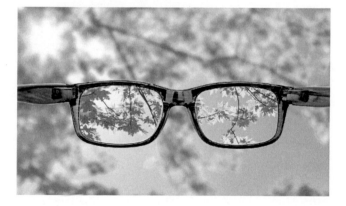

If you knew that you had a vision problem you could take steps to work around it (glasses). Otherwise you might compensate automatically in less desirable ways (squinting, or avoiding reading). Similarly, if you knew that your *mental* focus was blurry (due to ADHD) you could figure out some workarounds (medications, exercise, sleep hygiene). Otherwise you might be compensating automatically, and in less desirable ways (chronic stress).

*Would you want to know if your vision was impaired ?*

# 2

# What version of ADHD Do You Have?

Everyone's version of ADHD is unique but all versions are made up with different combinations of inattention, impulsivity, and restlessness. If your challenges are primarily with inattention and not so much impulsivity and restlessness, then you probably have inattentive ADHD. The old title for this version is ADD. If your challenges are more with impulsivity and restlessness, then you may have the restless/impulsive version. This used to be referred to as the hyperactive type. Some people struggle with all three. This is called the combined type. Today all versions are organized under the rubric of ADHD. Tomorrow, who knows?

## Inattention • Impulsivity • Restlessness

### Inattention
Distractible – sluggish processing – difficulties focusing and sustaining attention – disorganization – *low* working memory capacity.

### Impulsivity
Acting before thinking – interrupting others – blurting things out – difficulty delaying gratification.

### Restlessness (hyperactivity)
Motor is always running – hard to be still – can feel like an unstoppable lava flow.

# Obstacle

**How can you monitor ADHD when one of the symptoms of ADHD is poor self-monitoring?**

# Workaround

**Here is a structured exercise to help you monitor your executive functioning:**

Directions

1. Look the list of executive functions listed on page 30 (You may choose to copy and print the page so you can write on it).
2. Place a check in each box next to each ADHD symptom that fits you.
3. If you have symptoms not mentioned, add these to the list.
4. Review this list to make sure it fits.
5. Write down the three symptoms that cause you the most difficulty on a separate piece of paper.
6. Take the paper with you. Set your intention to notice when any of these symptoms *show up* during the day or week. Make note when they do. (*EG: If intolerance of boredom was what you selected, then try to notice whenever you are bored, or trying not to be bored. If you can log it somehow this will help you remember it*).
7. If you have trouble following these directions, then write *"difficulty following directions"* as your first symptom.

# 2 Obstacle

**You need a dual focus of attention in order be able to recognize (and then work around) ADHD.**

A dual focus of attention involves simultaneously monitoring your inner and outer worlds.

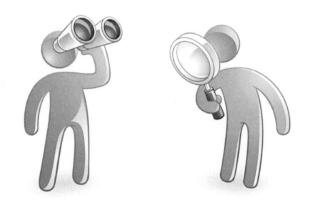

# Workaround

**Practice mindful self-monitoring.**

Mindful self-monitoring involves focusing inwardly on the activities of your mind. The goal is awareness, not change. Meditation is a form of mindful self-monitoring.

*Practice mindful self-monitoring.*

# Obstacle

You don't believe that you are disciplined enough to start a meditation practice.

# Workaround

**5-10 minutes per day of meditation will change your mind.**
You can restore your faith in your ability to stick with it by approaching meditation in an ADHD-friendly way. Make it as easy as possible to get a toehold. Do you think you could realistically commit to 5 or 10 minutes per day? You can listen to guided meditations or follow a structure, like focusing on breath. You don't have to sit on a pillow. Yes, this is mental exercise, but the gym can be wherever you are.

*5-10 minutes per day of meditation*
*will change your mind.*

**2**

# 2 Obstacle

**Judgment can be so deeply engrained in you that it is hard to recognize.** The problem with judgment is that it is often served up as kernels of truth wrapped in layers of negative bias. Many people with ADHD are so used to listening to judgment that it feels like breathing air. It may be judgment itself that is making you feel bad, not your ADHD.

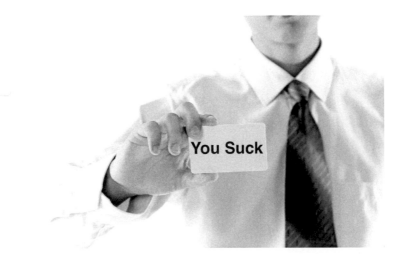

# Workaround

**You can un-invite judgment.**
You cannot control whether we have ADHD, but you can control whether you allow judgment into your home as a mental guest!

## *You can un-invite judgment.*

# How to un-invite judgment

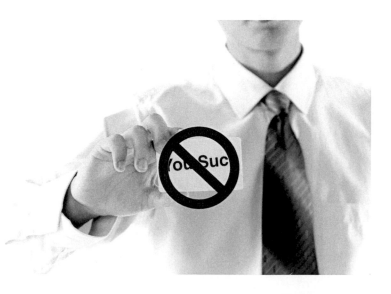

- Notice judgment each time it appears
- Label it, "judgment"
- Remind self that judgment is not OK
- Re-direct your attention elsewhere
- Repeat above steps
  (1,000 times per day if necessary)

# 2

# Obstacle

Impulsive, restless, and distractible people don't seem like good candidates for meditation.

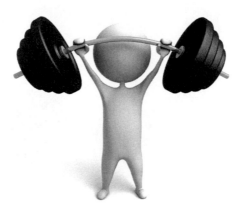

# Workaround

**Wrong! Impulsive/restless/distractible people may be the best candidates for meditation.**

We get the most practice exercising our attention muscles. We are easily distracted. The very act of noticing when your mind drifts (and gently bringing it back) is what strengthens your attention muscle. Each time you refocus your attention you execute one repetition. Think of lifting weights. *More reps mean bigger muscles.* The practice of meditation is **not** about emptying your mind. It is about actively monitoring the activities of your mind and directing your attention (with intention) to your breath, or wherever you choose.

*Impulsive/restless/distractible people may be the best candidates for meditation.*

# Monitoring Experiment

2

This is an experiment to help you recognize, without judgment, what happens as you intend to get started on a goal-directed activity. Whether you actually get started is not as important as the information you gather about what happens.

**1. Pick a goal** involving something you wish to accomplish this week (e.g.: composing an email, calling someone, cleaning or maintaining something). Write this goal on a piece of paper.

**2. Observe** (without judgment) what happens when you try to get started. For example: If you procrastinate, notice how you procrastinate. If you set an alarm do you ignore it? If so, how many times? How do treat yourself if you fail to get started when you think you should? Are you hard on yourself? Are you feeling frustration, shame, guilt, and stress? Notice if the task looms larger the longer you avoid it.

**3. Label** everything you observe. If you notice yourself avoiding getting started then label this as *avoidance* or *procrastination*. If you are stressing as you attempt to start then label this in your mind as, *"I am stressing when I think about getting started."*

4. **Debrief** by looking at the process as a whole at the end of the week. Write down patterns that you noticed. Once you can recognize predictable patterns, you can begin to figure out ways to work around them.

**2**

# Chapter 2 Summary
# Recognizing ADHD

**Recognition involves mindfully monitoring patterns of living without necessarily modifying them.** Monitoring can certainly lead to modifying, but it is important to treat these as separate steps. Sometimes people get stuck and feel unable to change because then have combined monitoring and modifying into one big, clunky step.

Mindfulness is about paying attention to the present moment without judgment. For our purposes, mindfulness and recognition are synonymous. Meditation practices develop the mindfulness/recognition *muscles*. When meditating, you notice when your mind has wandered, label where it went, and bring your attention back to the present. It has to do with observing (not emptying) your mind. I recommend that you find a way to develop a regular meditation practice. Meditation will not only enhance your capacity to recognize your ADHD, but may also help you learn to not take ADHD personally.

Recognizing patterns, without having to do something to change them enables you to relax, unclench, and consider your options. Naming (labeling) the activities of your mind is an effective way to tame them.

You can work around your ADHD when you can recognize it and anticipate its influence. You will be less likely to be taken by surprise by your executive *under*-functioning when you know how your symptoms are predictable. For example, the other day someone started giving me complex directions that would have required me to remember a sequence of left and right turns. I realized that there was no way I would be able to remember these directions (due to my ADHD). I interrupted the person and asked him to skip the directions and just give the address so I could plug it into my GPS navigator. I arrived at the destination without incident. Hurray!

The next step leading to the integration of ADHD is acceptance. Accepting ADHD is acknowledgment that having ADHD is not a choice.

# Chapter 3

# Accepting ADHD

Reframing and recognizing ADHD are precursors to accepting it. Acceptance is a separate step. It is not uncommon for adults with ADHD to reframe and recognize ADHD, but still not accept it in themselves. Some people get stuck here. You may have some very negative personal meanings associated with acceptance like, "I don't want to accept that I am defective," or "I'm a fighter, and I'm not going to surrender to this." The concept of acceptance has become contaminated. Acceptance does not imply approval. Acceptance is essentially acknowledging what is. Ironically, denying ADHD (when it is actually present) can wreak the greatest havoc because ADHD doesn't work around itself.

This chapter will highlight workarounds for each of the following obstacles to acceptance:
- You think that it is wimpy to *give in* and accept ADHD without a fight
- Your ADHD can't be cured or defeated but you don't want to admit it
- Trying harder only makes your ADHD symptoms worse
- Unrealistic (*wannabe*) expectations are a setup for failure
- The cost of living is higher when you have ADHD
- The notion of accepting ADHD can seem depressing to you
- You think that you have to like ADHD in order to accept it
- You continue having difficulties accepting ADHD

# 3 Obstacle

**You think that is wimpy to *give in* and accept ADHD without a fight.**

# Workaround

**The idea of fighting ADHD doesn't even make sense, as there is nothing to fight.**

ADHD is not an entity with a will. It is a neurological disorder, not the local bully. It takes courage to accept what is.

*It takes courage to accept what is.*

# Obstacle

**Trying harder only makes your symptoms worsen.**

# Workaround

***Relax into your strength.***

If you have ever taken a yoga class you may have been invited to, "relax into your strength." This is because optimal functioning, or integration, is associated with relaxation, not tension. The act of trying harder is likely to make the symptoms of ADHD worse. Trying harder can make you tense (rigid). Relaxing into strength may not be an intuitive approach, but it is an effective stance for working around your ADHD.

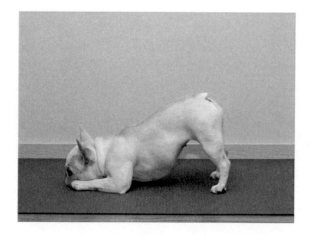

*Relax into your strength.*

# 3 Obstacle

**You tend to do things the hard way even though an easier way is available.**
Unrealistic expectations are *wannabe expectations* because they are based on how you *wannabe*, not how you actually are. *Wannabe expectations* (EG: expecting yourself to perform like a normal person) may be a greater source of suffering than ADHD itself. The reason may be that unrealistic expectations almost inevitably result in performance failures, and chronic performance failures can cascade into despair, demoralization and depression.

# Workaround

**Determine if this is an acceptance or an automaticity problem.**
Either you haven't fully accepted the fact that you have a disability (ADHD), or you have accepted your disability but you haven't fully retrofitted the automated routines that you rely on with ADHD workarounds. The latter is an automaticity problem.

1. Acceptance problem: ADHD is considered significant enough to be covered by the American with Disabilities Act. That makes ADHD a 300lb gorilla. It usually doesn't pay to ignore 300lb gorillas. However, the guy on crutches (on the next page) may be taking the stairs (vs. the elevator) to demonstrate how he is un-phased by his disability (gorilla). He believes that he can over-ride his disability by acting as if there is no gorilla. Are you like the guy on crutches who would rather suffer than accept that he has a disability?

2. Automaticity problem: Even though you have accepted your ADHD you still need to examine and *ADHD-proof* the myriad of automated routines that you rely on to make sure that they are ADHD-friendly. You may be working harder to the extent that the routines that you have on autopilot were founded on the assumption of your normality. If you are accustomed to doing things the hard way, you might be like the guy on crutches taking the stairs simply because he has always taken the stairs. He never even noticed that there was an elevator.

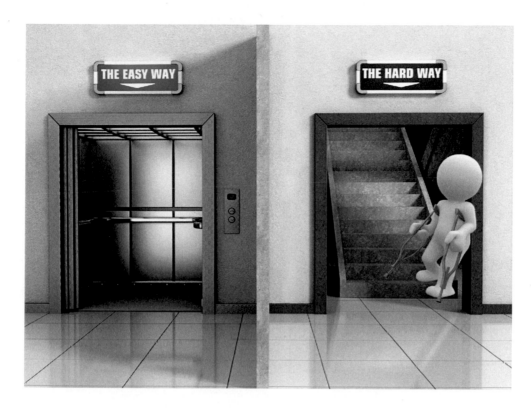

**Top Ten Reasons why the guy on crutches is choosing the stairs over of the elevator:**

10. He doesn't want to use the elevator as a crutch.
9. He wants to be normal, so he's not going to "give in" to the elevator.
8. "Crutches? Are you referring to these armpit extensions?"
7. There are bad men (also on crutches) who are chasing him.
6. He's renting the crutches so he wants to be sure to get his money's worth.
5. He has a fear of falling (and not being able to get back up) while in the elevator.
4. He takes *climbing the corporate ladder* way too literally.
3. He is worried about *elevator addiction*.
2. Crutches don't leave a carbon footprint.
1. What elevator?

# 3 Obstacle

**You don't want to admit that your ADHD can't be cured or defeated.**

# Workaround

**You are actually empowered by admitting your powerlessness over ADHD.**
Although ADHD is not an addiction, the first step toward health is the same as it
is with addictions. This involves admitting powerlessness over what you can't
control. Admitting powerless over ADHD is what allows you to work around it.

---

*The Serenity Prayer*

God (or higher power)
Grant me the serenity
To accept the things I cannot change
The courage to change the things I can
And the wisdom to know the difference

---

# Obstacle

**ADHD is expensive!**

# Workaround

Accept that **the cost of living is just higher if you have ADHD.**

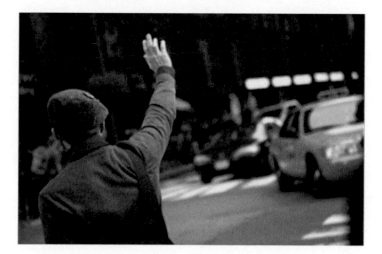

"I always leave my hat in a cab when I travel to NYC. I don't feel bad about it anymore. Now I bring at least two hats when I travel to New York since I know that I will be saying goodbye to at least one of them." (Author)

*The cost of living is just higher*
*if you have ADHD.*

# 3 Obstacle

**The idea of accepting ADHD seems depressing.**

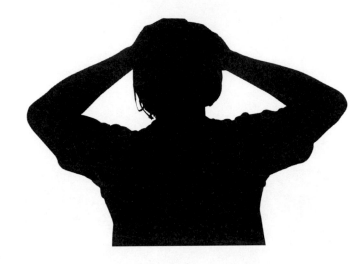

# Workaround

**Denial leaves you exposed to risk without protection.**
People who say that the idea of accepting their ADHD is depressing are probably anticipating depression. They won't find out until they actually accept their ADHD that it is actually just the opposite. It is so much more depressing to repeatedly bang your head against the wall while hoping for a different outcome. Acceptance enables you to integrate *what is* and thus work around obstacles.

*Denial leaves you exposed to risk without protection.*

# Obstacle

3

You confuse acceptance with approval.

# Workaround

**Acceptance is not the same as approval.**
Accepting ADHD is a separate issue from how you feel about it. You can accept it and hate it at the same time. I hate paying taxes, but I accept that I will inevitably have to pay them.

*Acceptance is not the same as approval.*

# 3 Obstacle

You continue having difficulties accepting ADHD. You are stuck here.

# Workaround

**Acceptance is so fundamental to taking control that it is important that you identify and address whatever is making acceptance a tough pill to swallow.** This is not the step to skip over! This could be a good time to reach out to an ADHD knowledgeable professional to help you untangle the web of meanings, associations, and memories that may be linked to your reluctance to accept your ADHD.

*This is not the step to skip over!*

3

# Chapter 3 Summary
# Accepting ADHD

To accept what is, is to align expectations with the way things are. Denial, however, is more likely to involve aligning expectations with how you wish things were. Denial involves a lot of extra work (like the guy with a sprained ankle routinely taking the stairs instead of the elevator). Acceptance, however, enables you to integrate *the way things are* into patterns of daily living EG: recognizing that, when you are on crutches, the elevator is a better option than the stairs. Although the act of accepting *the way things are* can be painful, it usually leads to a greater sense of control. Acceptance makes life easier because it means going with, not against, the flow.

Having ADHD (but not accepting it) can make your life far more difficult than it needs to be. One strong argument for accepting ADHD is simply the fact that you will still have the disorder whether you accept or deny it. Accepting ADHD enables you to align your self expectations with your actual capacities which, in turn, increases the likelihood of success. Unrealistic expectations increase the odds of failure and demoralization. Letting go of unrealistic expectations involves tolerating some losses, however. It might be a loss to let go of the belief that you can overcome your organizational obstacles by trying harder. It might be a loss to let go of the hope that some day you will be *normal*.

What do you do if you find yourself having trouble accepting your ADHD? If you have worked on accepting your ADHD but still find yourself stuck, then you might congratulate yourself. It is crucial that you noticed this! Acceptance is so fundamental to taking control that it is important that you identify and address whatever is making acceptance a tough pill to swallow. This is not the step to skip over! This could be a good time to reach out to a professional to help you untangle the web of meanings, associations, and memories that may be linked to your reluctance to accept your ADHD.

# Chapter 4

# Setting ADHD-friendly Goals

The act of deliberately transforming an imagined potential into a reality begins with setting goals. People with ADHD face significant challenges when it comes to constructing and realizing goals. Despite your best intentions, boredom, distraction, and working memory glitches can derail you. You can become mired in detail such that you lose track of your goal altogether. This chapter will highlight some ADHD-friendly workarounds for the obstacles below:

- Goals that are undefined or vague
- Goals that are out of sight (& thus out of mind)
- Goals that are boring
- Goals that are negative

# 4 Obstacle

**Your goals are vague.**
Amorphous goals lead to amorphous outcomes. They are not motivating. "I am going to fly airplanes" is vague.

# Workaround

**Make your goals specific.**
Define them explicitly. Name them. Say them out loud. Write them down. Tell someone. Well-defined goals have higher success rates and are more intrinsically motivating. "I am going to get my pilot's license and get a job flying commercial jets," is more specific.

*Well-defined goals have higher success rates.*

# Obstacle

4

**You can easily lose sight of your goals.**
Once the initial spark of creativity subsides it is easy for people with ADHD to lose track of goals. Resonating goals can be intrinsically motivating, but they must be remembered. Goals can be hard to remember since they exist (*out of sight*) in the projected future. *Out of sight, out of mind* is an ADHD thing.

# Workaround

**Externalize your goals**
Create symbolic representations of your goals and place them strategically in your environment. You might display them on a white-board or on the bathroom mirror. You won't need to try to remember your goals when they are literally in your face.

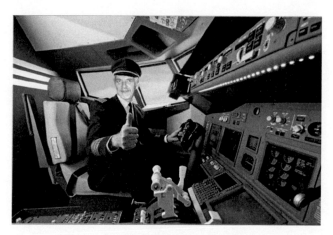

*If your goal is to become a commercial jet pilot:*
1. *Look for a stock photo of a pilot sitting in a cockpit of a jet.*
2. *Edit the image by superimposing a photo of your own head over the pilot's head.*
3. *Display the image prominently.*

# 4 Obstacle

**You tend to fail reaching goals which are intrinsically boring.**

# Workaround

**You can workaround boredom by pairing a bland goal with an activity that is fun or interesting.** Once linked, the fun activity can help energize and sustain your attention along the pathway to an uninteresting goal.

Below is an example of a paired workaround using exercise and fun.

> Frank was unable to get to the gym consistently. He loved to play basketball, however, so he decided to join a basketball league at the park. He got into shape simply by playing in the league. He was also motivated to lift weights in order to improve his game. Frank harnessed his love of basketball as well as the structure that the league provided to pull him toward his goal of getting get in shape, and he did it without really trying.

# Obstacle

4

**You set negative goals.**
When the goal involves avoiding something or preventing something from happening the goal is a *negative goal*. For example, "I am going stop losing friends," is a negative goal. Negative goals are associated with anxiety. If you succeed in preventing something from happening your only reward will be relief.

# Workaround

**Make sure that your goals involve moving toward something.**
When the goal is to make something happen, or to take on a challenge, it is a positive goal. An example of a positive goal might be, "I am going to make two new friends." When you set goals that involve moving toward something, the reward circuitry in your brain will be stimulated. *Yummy* dopamine will be released. Although facing a challenge may still be very difficult, it is likely to be rewarding because you are facing it.

*Make sure that your goals involve moving toward something.*

**4**

# Chapter 4 Summary
# Setting ADHD-friendly Goals

The acts of reframing, recognizing, and accepting ADHD are foundational but they don't necessarily move you forward. In order to move forward and intentionally turn a potential into a reality you need a goal. Unfortunately, people with ADHD face some significant obstacles when it comes to realizing goals. We are as infamous for not realizing our ideas (turning potentials into realities) as we are famous for coming up with lots of new ideas. It is important that you attend to goal-setting mindfully. Your future is at stake! Goals are what enable you to intentionally define your own future. Indeed, if you don't actively define your intended future it will likely be defined for you! Modify your goal-setting strategies in order to ensure that they are ADHD-friendly. The subjects in the success and ADHD studies did.

The probability that you will successfully attain your goal **decreases** when:
- Goals are undefined or vague
- Goals are out of sight (& thus out of mind)
- Goals are boring
- Goals are negative (avoidant)

The probability that you will successfully attain your goal **increases** when:
- Goals are well defined
- Goals are externalized
- Goals are paired with fun
- Goals involve moving toward (vs. avoiding) something

# Chapter 5

# Managing Morale

Morale is associated with energy, mood, drive, agency, motivation, timing, and quality of life. In the military, morale is related to the will to fight. For us, morale is related to the will to keep working around obstacles until we reach our goals. For people already facing an uphill struggle with ADHD, moral can be the deciding resilience factor.

In this chapter you will discover some workarounds for the following morale related obstacles:

- You feel beaten down and demoralized by ADHD
- You aren't used to paying attention to your morale
- You are still troubled by memories of being demoralized in the past
- Chronic stress is bad for your morale
- Keeping your energy up can be difficult when there are many (often boring) steps on the path toward a goal
- You have difficulties staying motivated

# 5 | Obstacle

You feel beaten down and demoralized by ADHD.

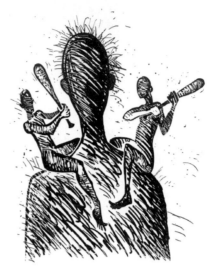

# Workaround

**ADHD cannot demoralize you. If you feel demoralized, it is probably due to something you have control over.** Below are some possible sources of demoralization to be curious about.

- How you take care of yourself
- How you motivate yourself
- How forgiving you are of yourself
- How you show up as your own friend
- Who you listen to

*ADHD cannot demoralize you. If you feel demoralized, it is probably due to something you have control over.*

# Obstacle

**You aren't used to paying attention to your morale.**

# Workaround

**Here is an exercise to help you monitor your morale.**

Directions: Set your intention to notice how you take care of yourself. The questions below can serve as a guide.

- How do you tend to treat yourself when you make mistakes?
- Would you be comfortable treating someone else this way?
- How do you tend to treat yourself when you succeed? EG: Do you give yourself credit where credit is due?
- Do you give yourself as much credit as you do criticism? (What is the ratio)?

*How do you tend to treat yourself when you make mistakes?*

5

# 5 Obstacle

**You are haunted by memories of being demoralized in the past.**

# Workaround

**Send your *past self* some empathy.**

Now that you know something about ADHD you can make better sense of the challenges you faced earlier in your life. This exercise offers you a chance to send your *past self* some warmth and empathy. You can even boost your morale in a memory. Try this exercise below only if you are comfortable exploring these memories. If you feel you are not ready, please stop.

> **Think of any ADHD-related incident that occurred when you were young such that, when you remember it, you still feel a little bad about it.** Perhaps you felt like giving up after dropping the ball on something, or you were scattered at a time when it was important to be focused. Maybe you were embarrassed about forgetting something important. Someone may have made fun of you for being *spacey*. Did you assume that you were irresponsible or lazy, etc?
>
> **Picture your *past self* in that scene.**
> Imagine speaking warmly to your *past self* (privately or out loud).
> Start sentences with the phrase, "No wonder…"
> EG: "No wonder it is so hard for you to sit still in school. You have ADHD," or, "No wonder you are so overwhelmed. You try so hard, yet you end up late because you don't know that you have ADHD. "The empathy is in the "No wonder you……."
>
> **Now picture how your *past self* responds to the warmth and empathy.** This memory has been altered.

# Obstacle

**You get stingy when it comes to giving yourself credit.**
Do you tend to discount the importance of small steps that you make? (EG: You withhold giving yourself credit until you have completed your goal.)

# Workaround

**Acknowledge any effort that you make, no matter how small.**
Since tiny accomplishments can still involve high degrees of difficulty (especially for the organizationally impaired) it is important that you give yourself credit (where credit is due). This is a resilience factor that is within your control.

Try the experiment below to experience how savoring credit can affect you:

1.  Write down any three things that you expended any energy on today, no matter how small.
2.  Look at them one at a time.
3.  Take a few breaths as you savor each one.
4.  Notice how it feels to allow yourself to savor your efforts.
5.  At the end of the day, write down everything you expended any energy on all day (no matter how small). Include anything you might tend to take for granted like parenting, chores, or going to work. Even contemplating something counts.
6.  As you savor this list, notice whether the energy level in your body matches the efforts you expended and acknowledged.

# 5 Obstacle

Keeping your energy up can be difficult when there are many (often boring) steps on the path toward a goal.

# Workaround

**Have fun!**

Protect your morale by making sure you are having fun whenever possible. Spice up the path with what makes you smile. Listen to music. Make up a game. Fun is an essential strategy for sustaining attention.

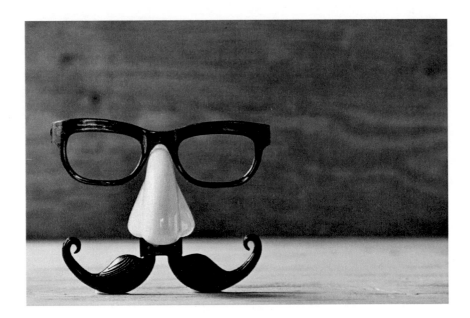

*Have fun!*

# Obstacle

**5**

**You have difficulties with self-motivation.**

We are better able to maintain higher levels of motivation at the beginning (idea) stage of a project. However, we can easily lose that motivation during the later stages. Motivational styles matter when considering their impact over time. EG: Negative motivation (stress, harshness, fear) for example, may be effective motivators in the short term, but harmful in the long term. It is useful to monitor your motivational style. Once you can monitor it, you can fine-tune it.

# Workaround

**Notice how you tend to motivate yourself.**

**Directions**: Try to pay attention to how you motivate yourself (using the question provided below). The goal is to observe, not change. It might be helpful to write the question down and stick it in your pocket as a reminder. It would be ideal to keep a log.

• Do you motivate yourself with stress?
• Do you encourage yourself?
• Do you acknowledge your progress to yourself?
• Do you tend to play to win or not to lose?
• Do you tend to motivate yourself positively or negatively?
• Do you tend to push or pull yourself toward goals?

*Do you motivate yourself with stress?*

# Chapter 5 Summary
# Managing Morale

Morale is associated with will, desire, meaning, confidence, and motivation. When morale is high we are more likely to believe in our ability to realize our goals. When moral is low, we might feel like giving up rather than persisting.

Morale is related to how we take care of ourselves as well as how we motivate ourselves. People with ADHD can be particularly vulnerable to de-moralization. If you have ADHD it is especially important that you monitor and protect your morale. When you advocate for, and are kind to yourself, you are protecting your morale.

Motivational states are like battery packs supplying the energy we need to move forward toward a goal-directed future. Motivational states provide the energy to overcome obstacles and to delay gratification. People with ADHD have an impaired ability to picture the intended future while simultaneously engaging with boring details in the present. The inability to sustain motivation can drain your batteries and lower your morale.

Protect your morale by taking charge of keeping yourself motivated. You can do this by building motivation into systems of organization, externalizing big picture goals, and building fun into action plans, for example.

I have come across many people with ADHD caught in a cycle of trying and failing. I remember someone telling me, "You can only hit your head against the wall so many times before you give up." This is what it means to be demoralized. The problem is that the majority of these people assumed that they were demoralized because they had ADHD.

Demoralization is not a symptom of ADHD! It is more likely the result of doing what doesn't work over and over again. Ultimately your morale will suffer if you are expecting yourself to get over your ADHD and function like a normal person. Your morale will be enhanced each time you work around your ADHD.

Chapter 6

# Finding ADHD-friendly Pathways to Action

Pathways to action are the means by which you get to your goal. These means involve methods, strategies, and systems of organization. "To dos" are pathways to action. Even If your goal is to enjoy a relaxing vacation in Hawaii you will still have to manage lots of details before you can unpack your flip-flops.

People with ADHD need specialized pathways. You may be failing to reach your goals because you are attempting to follow the same pathways that normal people use without modifying them to make them ADHD-friendly.

- Pathways can become slippery slopes
- A common error made by people with ADHD is to take on too much at once
- You can set yourself up for failure by following ADHD-unfriendly pathways to action
- Your brain is organizationally challenged
- To-do lists can be very useful. They can also become oppressive and de-motivational
- Your mind is susceptible to being organized by the external environment

# 6 Obstacle

**Pathways to action can turn into slippery slopes.**
It is risky to follow a pathway to action without determining whether or not it is ADHD-friendly. Pathways to action are fraught with challenges for people with ADHD. We are at risk of becoming mired in the details involved with the pathway such that we lose track of the destination.

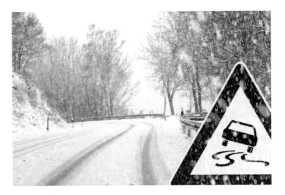

# Workaround

**Make sure that pathways to action are ADHD-friendly or can modified to become ADHD-friendly.**

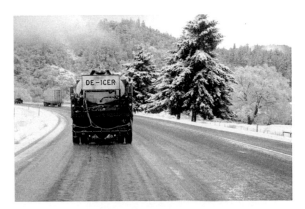

# Obstacle

**6**

**A common error made by people with ADHD is to take on too much at once.**

# Workaround

**Try to bite off less than you can chew.**
See if you can do less than you think you are capable of. This may be harder than you think.

*Try to bite off less than you can chew.*

# 6 Obstacle

**You are more likely to fail when following pathways designed for normal people.**

You may be setting yourself up for failure by relying on ADHD-unfriendly pathways.

*For example, normal people can innately estimate the amount of time it will take to get ready for something. People with ADHD who rely on their innate ability to know how much time it will take to get ready for something are probably going to be late and/or unprepared.*

# Workaround

**Adapt pathways to action so they are ADHD-friendly.**

ADHD-friendly pathways increase the likelihood of success.

An ADHD-friendly adaptive strategy: *Automatically add 15 minutes to whatever your innate time estimation for getting ready is.* Use the five processes below to create ADHD-friendly pathways to action:

- Automation – Set up systems that can run themselves.
- Navigation – Use smart devices with GPS.
- Externalization – Plant cues in your environment.
- Habituation – You don't have to remember a habit.
- Strategy – Use your mind to work around your ADHD-addled brain.

# Obstacle

6

**Your brain is organizationally challenged.**
It starts to hurt when you push it.

# Workaround

**Take the pressure off your brain by allowing ADHD-friendly systems of organization to carry the load.**
When you develop systems that compensate for your ADHD, you take the pressure off your organizationally challenged brain. Optimal systems are self-sustaining.

EG:    A system for where you leave your keys.
A system for remembering passwords.
A system for keeping track of your schedule.
A system for going to bed.
A system for getting exercise.
A system for storing your shoes.
A system for just about everything.

*Take the pressure off your brain by building
ADHD-friendly systems of organization
to carry the load.*

# 6 Obstacle

**It is difficult to focus (internally) on your own private thoughts for very long.**
ADHD impairs your natural ability to hold information in mind. Your attention is vulnerable to being hijacked at any time by random shiny objects in the physical environment. This can interfere with your capacity to utilize foresight and/or hindsight as resources as you navigate the pathways to your goal.

# Workaround

**Externalize your thoughts**
You can use your sensitivity to the external world to your advantage by peppering your environment with information that you need to know (but might forget). Plant this information in your physical world for your future self to *discover*. Write inspirational messages on your bathroom mirror. Send yourself an email. Purchase white boards and use them to organize your thoughts. Give a presentation on something that you wish to pursue just for the purpose of externalizing and developing your thoughts. Talk to yourself (out loud) whenever possible so you can hear your thoughts.

*Talk to yourself (out loud) whenever possible so you can hear your thoughts.*

# Obstacle

**6**

To-do lists can be very useful ways to organize pathways to action. They can also become oppressive if they are too long.

# Workaround

**Create short TO-DO lists.**
No more than 5 items at a time. Write down 3-5 things you wish to accomplish in a day and carry the list with you.

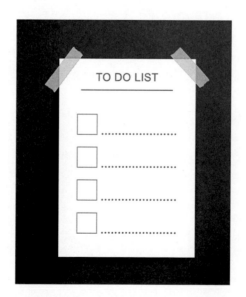

*Create short TO-DO lists.*

**6**

# Chapter 6 Summary
# Finding ADHD-friendly Pathways to Action

Pathways to action help us get from A to B. Pathways to action refer to what we must do (or the path we must take) to reach our big picture goals. If your big-picture goal is to be a teacher in a public school, for example, a pathway to action will involve enrolling in school and earning a teaching credential.

Since pathways to action can be slippery, it is important to be mindful about how we construct them. Pathways to action tend to be detail oriented, so people with ADHD are at risk of getting lost in the details. We can easily become overwhelmed and flooded by *too much information* and lose the linkage between the big-picture goal and the pathway to action. One solution involves shortening to-do lists. Think of how you feel when you look at a big, long to-do list. A big to-do list can be overwhelming.

It is important to be mindful of the pathways to action that we choose to get to our goals. We must be sure that our pathways to action are ADHD-friendly. This is where we really must separate ourselves from normal people. People who have ADHD, but haven't integrated it, may find themselves crashing because the pathways they have are ADHD-unfriendly. In other words, they set the bar too high.

ADHD-friendly pathways to action build in compensatory measures that address the challenges posed by inattention, impulsivity, and restlessness. These usually involve keeping it simple. For example, when using a "to-do list," be sure that the list is small (3-5 items). Take baby steps and lower the bar of expectations. It is better to take on less than what you think you can handle and be successful than to push yourself to your breaking point and crash. ADHD-friendly pathways to action can also be externalized by structuring the external environment with prompts cues and reminders.

# Chapter 7

# Finding Creative Solutions

Apopular belief holds that people with ADHD are more creative people. Is this true? No. We are not more creative or gifted than the rest of the population. We have difficulty following directions so we re-invent the wheel regularly. We have gotten used to being creative out of necessity. We simply can't do most things the way that they are "supposed" to be done, thus we are well practiced at improvising. In this chapter we offer workarounds for the following creativity-oriented obstacles:

- You can't seem to do things the conventional way
- People with ADHD can arrive at accurate conclusions without being able to explain up how they got there
- You undervalue the idiosyncratic way that you solve problems
- By **not** knowing about the left hemisphere, you may limit the range of your workarounds
- By **not** knowing about the right hemisphere, you may limit the range of your workarounds

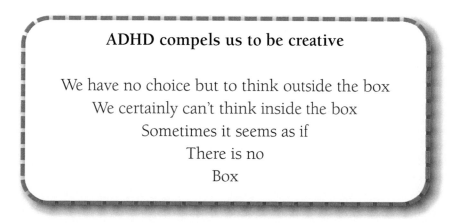

**ADHD compels us to be creative**

We have no choice but to think outside the box
We certainly can't think inside the box
Sometimes it seems as if
There is no
Box

# 7 Obstacle

**You can't seem to do things the conventional way.**

# Workaround

**Do it your own (bleeping) way!**
Unconventional methods may be more effective for creating pathways to action that are resonating (no matter how strange they may seem to others). *The proof is in the pudding!* If it helps you to write reminders on you bathroom mirror with lipstick, then write reminders on your bathroom mirror with lipstick. If it is easier to assemble something without looking at the directions, then assemble it without looking at the directions.

## *Do it your own (bleeping) way!*

# Obstacle

**You are self-conscious about being different.**
You don't want people to think you are weird so you try to pass for normal.

# Workaround

**Celebrate (*don't rehabilitate*) your idiosyncrasies.**
You are weird.  Embrace it!  Your uniqueness is your contribution.

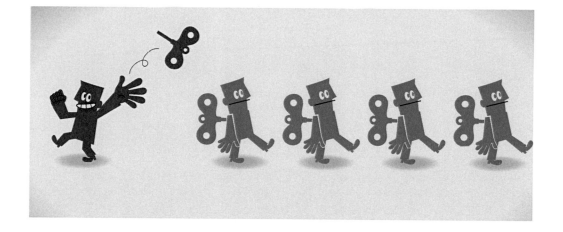

*Celebrate (don't rehabilitate) your idiosyncrasies.*

# 7 Obstacle

The range of your workarounds may by limited by what you don't know about the right hemisphere.

# Workaround

Knowing how your right hemisphere processes information can enhance your workarounds.

**Right hemisphere**
The big picture hemisphere is non-linear and impressionistic.

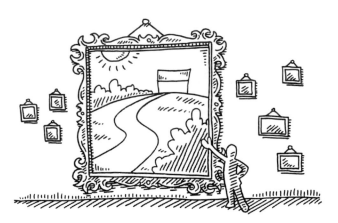

  Do you ever find yourself knowing answers without knowing the steps that lead to those answers? You may have your right hemisphere to thank. This is because your right hemisphere processes information in a unique way (the right is not so impaired by ADHD). The right is more big-picture/holistic/subjective. The right hemisphere thinks via parallel distributed processing, which is a much more complex form of processing than serial processing (associated with the left). Consider the information that is conveyed in a picture (processed via the right), vs. 1,000 words of text (processed via the left).

# Obstacle

The range of your workarounds may by limited by what you don't know about the left hemisphere.

# Workaround

Knowing how your left hemisphere processes information can enhance your workarounds.

### Left hemisphere

The 1,000 words hemisphere is detail-oriented and particular.

The left hemisphere seems to be more adversely impacted by ADHD than the right. We have more trouble with serial processing, which is the form of thinking associated with the left hemisphere. The left hemisphere is linear, logical and linguistic. The left hemisphere tries to make sense of things. In particular, the left tries to make sense of the right hemisphere. Structure and organization are associated with the left. Conceptualizations and meanings begin in the right, but are articulated by the left. The dorsal-lateral prefrontal cortex has been associated with working memory and is located in the left hemisphere. People with ADHD are challenged with working memory deficits. Working memory is what enables us to remember (or not) who we are calling while we are dialing a phone number. While the right hemisphere tends to hold the big picture, the gist, or the whole, the left hemisphere holds the details. This is why we are referring to the left as the *1,000 words hemisphere* and the right as the *big picture hemisphere*. You can process complex information through parallel distributed processing (PDP) via imagery, and other forms of symbolic representations primarily through the right hemisphere, or you can try to codify the same information using words. As you can imagine, much is lost in translation. Think of the difference between gazing first hand at the painting of the Mona Lisa vs. having someone describe what it looks like in words. People with ADHD often have difficulty following directions. This may be because directions are usually linear and are the byproduct of serial processing. This may be why, when figuring out how to assemble something, many people with ADHD will skip the directions all together and just look at all the parts to see how they might fit together. We can easily become overwhelmed by details. In fact it would be quite an accomplishment if you got this far reading all of these words describing the left hemisphere if you have ADHD. The author decided to design this book to be more right hemisphere friendly by reducing the amount of text (except in this section) and increasing the amount of concepts that are in condensed into *gist* form.

**7**

# Obstacle

Many people with ADHD discount their uncanny ability to come up with accurate conclusions without knowing the steps that lead to those conclusions.

# Workaround

**Take advantage of your thinking advantage.**
Don't discount your thinking just because you can't explain the steps that lead to your conclusion. There evidence to support the legitimacy of this kind of problem solving. This anomaly may be best understood by examining the difference between the ways that each of our two cerebral hemisphere's process information (See previous pages).

# Chapter 7 Summary
# Finding Creative Solutions

Our institutions, schools and bureaucracies tend to favor more recursive, top-down, and rule-based approaches to problem solving. The successful people with ADHD in the Gerber study (like most people with ADHD), however, tended to utilize emergent, bottom-up, novel, and outside the box approaches to problem solving. Although our problem solving does tend to be more creative, it is not because we're born with creativity genes. We are more creative because we have to be creative out of necessity. The truth is that we are typically not so good at following convention. We cannot remember to follow rules consistently, and are frequently re-inventing the wheel. We are outliers who have become accustomed to making it up as we go. An accurate understanding of the differences between how the two cerebral hemispheres process information might shed some light on our apparent creativity. The right hemisphere processes multiple levels at once. Dreams, metaphors, and imagery are the byproducts of this kind of information processing. This is called parallel distributed processing (PDP). PDP is a non-linear, emergent form of thinking. The good news is that this form of thinking does not appear to be so compromised by ADHD. Parallel distributed processing is not sequential or logic based. PDP allows one to be able to jump to a conclusion correctly without necessarily following, or even knowing, the sequences that lead to that conclusion. Since serial processing appears to be more compromised for people with ADHD, we may have to rely on PDP more than the average person. We can learn how to harness and expand this right-brain power, as the ability to think outside the box can be a valuable trait in many contexts. A weakness in one area has lead to the strengthening of another. Some even refer to this as our, "spidey power."

The left hemisphere employs a linear, logical, and linguistic form of "thinking called serial processing (processing in sequences). This kind of thinking is more impaired with ADHD. Rules and directions involve serial processing. Although the world we live in tends to discount non-linear processing, it is important that we don't. Our operating system is different but valid. It can be an advantage, as people who are unconstrained by convention tend to come up with the new ideas. It is important to accept how you think. Whenever possible, do it your own (bleeping) way!

# Chapter 8

# Prioritizing Goodness of Fit

The ability to adapt the environment to oneself, and oneself to the environment was a factor shared in common by the successful adults with ADHD in the Gerber study. Essentially this means learning how to customize external environments to support your needs as well as adapting yourself to fit into environments that can't be overhauled. Since we with ADHD are especially susceptible to the influence of our environments, it pays to prioritize goodness of fit.

In this chapter you will find workarounds for the following goodness of fit obstacles:

- If the shoe doesn't fit…
- The world isn't set up for people with ADHD (or lefties)
- Sometimes people with ADHD choose environments that exaggerate their weaknesses and minimize their strengths
- It can be difficult for you to stay focused unless you find something interesting
- Many people with ADHD fear being trapped in boring environments
- Some adults with ADHD suffer more from being square pegs trying to fit into round holes than they do from having ADHD itself
- We have been dealt a poor hand (ADHD)
- Sometimes unconventional workarounds can seem strange and raise eyebrows

# 8 Obstacle

**The shoe doesn't fit...**

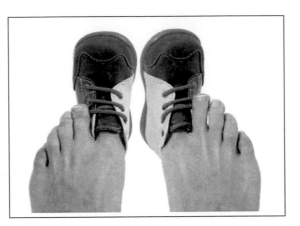

# Workaround

*...try on another shoe.*

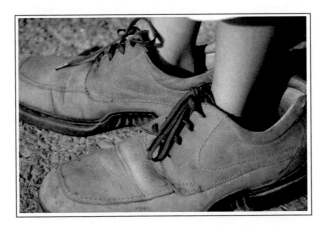

*If the shoe doesn't fit...try on another shoe.*

# Obstacle

8

**The world is not set up for people with ADHD (or left-handed people).**
Door handles, guitars, and place settings, etc. are usually configured for right-handed people. Lefties have to adapt far more than righties do. In a similar way the world is also set up for "normals" (those who don't have ADHD).

# Workaround

**Modify the external environment to match your needs as much as possible.**
In order to thrive, people with ADHD (like lefties) must figure out how to live in a world that is not designed for them.

For example: If you know that you'll never go to a gym consistently but you do want to work out, you could purchase the kinds of exercise equipment you use at the gym and build a gym in your house so you can exercise more consistently.

You could use a cabinet with glass windows as a dresser so you can see your clothes without having to open the drawer. You could put white boards throughout your house so you can capture thoughts and leave yourself reminders.

*Modify the external environment*
*to match your needs as much as possible.*

# 8 Obstacle

**Your chosen career path enhances your weaknesses more than your strengths.**

The environment you work in matters. You probably spend prime time hours there. A job that is tedious, detail oriented, and involves sitting still for long periods, for example, is not such a good match for someone with ADHD.

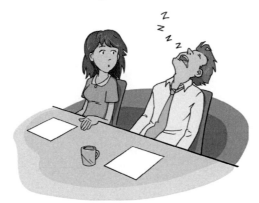

# Workaround

**Consider re-inventing yourself work-wise**

Find a job that rewards thinking outside the box. You are more likely to thrive as the idea person than the detail person.

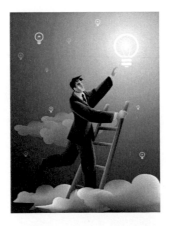

# Obstacle

**8**

**It can be difficult for you to stay focused unless you find something interesting.** The problem is that many things that you are doing are not that interesting.

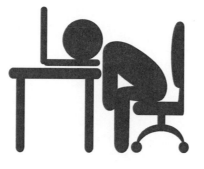

# Workaround

**Follow your Excitement!**

Follow your excitement wherever and whenever possible. When you are excited about something your attention system energizes and your focus improves. Pick activities or goals that really interest you. If you are stuck with something uninteresting, find a way to make it interesting enough by keeping yourself stimulated somehow.

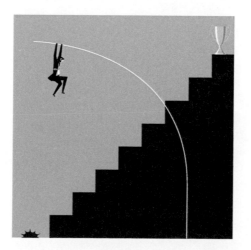

# 8 Obstacle

**You fear being trapped and bored.**
You dread waiting in lines, being on hold, and sitting through long meetings/classes.

# Workaround

**Bring entertainment with you as an insurance policy against boredom.**
Always carry some form of entertainment with you. Even waiting in line can be fun if you are playing a game on your handheld device. If you are able to pay closer attention by doodling or drawing when you are stuck in boring meetings or classes, then bring a "doodle notebook" with you.

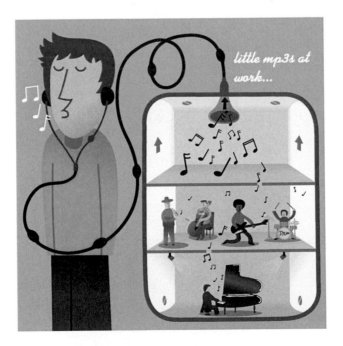

# Obstacle

You try to force yourself to fit in to mismatched environments and end up feeling like a square peg in a round hole.

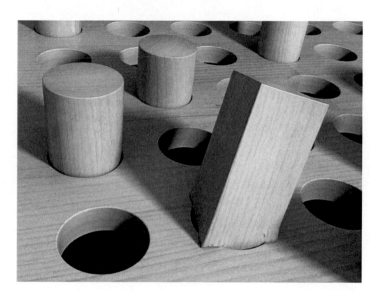

# Workaround

**It's Ok to be a square peg.  If possible, find a square hole.**
Having ADHD is hard enough. Why make life more difficult?   Place yourself in ADHD-friendly environments whenever possible.

# 8 | Obstacle

You have been dealt a poor hand (ADHD).

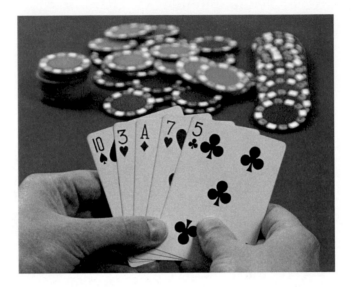

# Workaround

**Learn how to play a poor hand well.**

Play to your strengths. There are many strengths that people with ADHD share in common. These can be cultivated. Which of the strengths (listed below) apply to you. See if you can add to the list. How can you capitalize on these strengths?

**Some common strengths of people with ADHD:**
- Alert, focused, and stable in a crisis.
- Inventive (able to come up with new ideas/perspectives).
- Spontaneous. Fun to be around.
- Non-linear approach to problem solving.
- Practiced at letting go and moving on.
- Sensitive and intuitive.

# Obstacle

8

Sometimes unconventional workarounds can seem strange to people, and raise eyebrows.

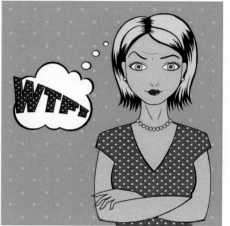

# Workaround

**Be willing to look like an idiot if that's what it takes to improve the quality of your life.**

The author was willing to look like an idiot. *For year and years I wore a fanny pack. It prevented me from losing my things. In fact I stopped losing things immediately. However, I was usually the only person in the room, or time zone, who was wearing a fanny pack. I decided that it was more important to stop losing things than it was to avoid looking like an idiot. Only recently,* I replaced my fanny pack with a messenger bag with a GPS gizmo attached to it.

*Be willing to look like an idiot if that's what it takes to improve the quality of your life.*

8

# Chapter 8 Summary
# Prioritizing Goodness of Fit

The successful adults with ADHD in the study were especially good at matching their environment with their personal attributes and their personal attributes with their environment. The result was a proper fit.

In order to create a good fit you must tune in to yourself. You need to gather information about your wants and needs. This is especially important for those of us with ADHD because the world is not set up for us. If our first move is to tune in to what the world (others) wants and needs from us, we will get out of synch with ourselves and become like a round peg trying to fit into a square hole. A good reference point to tune into is your own excitement. If you can identify what excites you, you can use your excitement to fuel your attention as well as give you direction. When in doubt, follow your excitement.

Try to match your environment to yourself if possible. For example, if you find yourself always doing office work in the kitchen, try moving your desk into the kitchen. If you are a student and you find that you study better at the coffee shop then go to the coffee shop to study. Pick environments that help you focus. (This doesn't necessarily mean the library).

If you are not able to match your environment with your needs then you can adapt yourself to the environment. For example, if you have to wait in a long line for something, you may want to bring entertainment with you to protect you from boredom. You really never have to be bored if you always have a podcast, a game, or a magazine, or some other form of entertainment with you. Ask yourself this question: What is more important, what works, or how it might look to others?

# Chapter 9

# Cultivating Supportive Relationships

Strong social connections are resilience factors. It can be soothing and inspiring to be in the company of other people, especially those who are working around their ADHD.

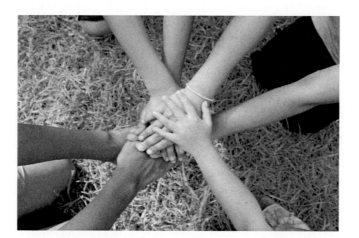

People with ADHD have some unique social challenges.

In this chapter you will find workarounds for the following relationship obstacles:

- Your chaotic mind is susceptible to being organized by the company that you keep
- You have lost faith in relationships because you keep getting *burned* by people after you trusted them
- You have ADHD and you are isolated
- You can easily become stuck/flooded/overwhelmed in the process of working around obstacles
- You can lose focus, drift, and waste time more easily when alone

# 9 Obstacle

You have lost faith in relationships because you have placed trust in people who have let you down.

# Workaround

**Trust is earned.**
Rethink how trust is acquired. Did those people earn your trust or was it gifted? Granting trust before it is earned is a good way to get hurt. What can you trust? You can trust what you observe and experience over time. You can trust what people do more than what people say. You can trust that whatever happens most of the time is likely to continue. EG: If someone promises to be on time (but is usually10 minutes late), you can trust that they will probably be 10 minutes late, no matter what they say.

*Trust is earned.*

# Obstacle

**9**

**Your chaotic mind is susceptible to becoming organized by the company that you keep.**

If you spend your time with judgmental people you will be challenged to walk away from them without feeling bad.

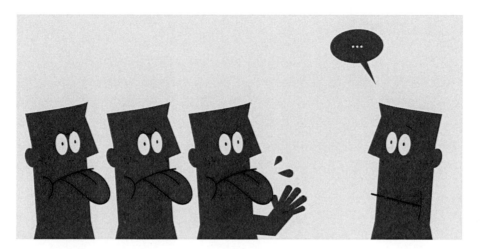

# Workaround

**Be picky about the company you keep.**

Hang out with people who accept you, appreciate you, don't judge you, respect you, and who enjoy being with you. Pick a mate carefully!

*Be picky about the company you keep.*

# 9 Obstacle

You have ADHD and you are socially isolated.

# Workaround

**Meet other people with ADHD.**
It can be a wonderful experience to be with people who understand what it is like to live with ADHD, because they too live with it. Many people with ADHD have not had the luxury of really knowing someone else with the disorder. Safe and supportive groups for people ADHD can be powerful sources of connection, inspiration, and motivation whenever there is a good fit. Support groups are listed on the ADDA website.

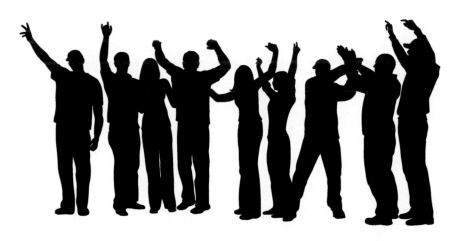

*Meet other people with ADHD.*

# Obstacle

You can become stuck, flooded, and overwhelmed trying to work around obstacles on your own.

# Workaround

Sometimes the best workaround is to ask for help, and then accept the help you have asked for.

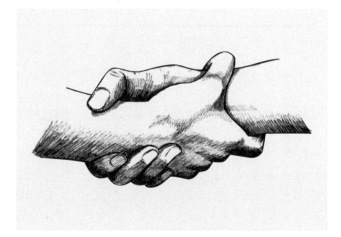

*Ask for help, and then
accept the help you have asked for.*

# 9 | Obstacle

**You can lose focus, drift, and waste time more easily when alone.**

# Workaround

**Even the passive presence of another person can provide enough structure to stabilize a chaotic mind.**

Some people with ADHD have found that just having a person sitting with them (doing nothing else) enables them to accomplish tasks that seemed overwhelming when the person wasn't sitting there. Go figure.

*Even the passive presence
of another person can provide enough structure
to stabilize a chaotic mind.*

**9**

# Chapter 9 Summary
# Cultivating Supportive Relationships

The successful adults in the study connected themselves with supportive people. None of them achieved success in isolation.

People with ADHD have some unique challenges in relationships. One challenge involves the way that our ADHD minds tend to be organized by the structure (environment) that we are in. Since a relationship is itself a structure, our minds are vulnerable to being organized by our relationships (for better or for worse). Thus we need to connect with people who accept us for who we are and support us, and we need protection from those who don't. One form of protection involves building trust (vs. gifting it). Building trust involves taking small risks and evaluating what happens next before taking more risks. In this way trust is earned. Taking big risks before trust is earned (gifting trust) is a setup to be hurt.

*Word on the street* is that we are not always so easy to live with. Although our ADHD is not exactly a relationship selling point, we do bring an exciting and somewhat unruly flavor to life. Some people find this attractive, others not so much. Try to partner with someone who finds this attractive. Once you do, be generous with your warmth and appreciation.

People with ADHD seem to be susceptible to getting stuck and overwhelmed. This may be the result of the neurological glitch that impairs our ability to plan and organize toward future goals. Asking for (and accepting) the right help is a powerful way to get unstuck (or to not get stuck in the first place). Impasses that seem intractable and insurmountable can sometimes melt away simply by getting the right help. We can make quantum leaps toward our goals when we ask for and utilize the right help.

I strongly recommend that you get to know other people who have ADHD. It can be uncanny to be with people who understand how you without you having to explain. Also, it can be validating that *you are not making this stuff* up when you see yourself in others.

# Chapter 10

# Practicing Persistence

The successful adults with ADHD in the study practiced persistence. Persistence is not related to gutting it out so much as it is to developing strategies that can make the journey more bearable. Of course you do want to make sure that you are persisting on a path that actually delivers you to your destination. Persistence doesn't help when you are persisting in the wrong direction. Impulsive, restless, and distractible people are more likely to give up prematurely. We must find workarounds that enable us to persist despite this tendency.

In the following chapter, you will find workarounds for the following persistence related challenges:

- The reason why you fail reach your goals is that you give up
- You pressure yourself to achieve success on the first try
- Persistence doesn't help when you are headed in the wrong direction
- You may compensate for ADHD by rushing yourself
- You are tempted to give up after becoming overwhelmed by the prospect of taking on some task

# 10 Obstacle

**The reason people with ADHD fail to reach their goals is often that they give up prematurely.**

# Workaround

**Don't Give Up.**
Work around obstacles until you succeed. If you really wish to accomplish your goal, the most important thing you can do is to not give up!

*Work around obstacles until you succeed.*

# Obstacle

Persistence doesn't help when you are headed in the wrong direction.

# Workaround

**If you're going to drive off into the sunset, make sure that you are heading west!** Make certain that your pathway to action actually leads to your destination.

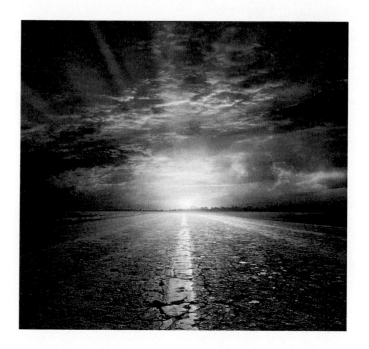

*If you're going to drive off into the sunset, make sure that you are heading west!*

# 10 Obstacle

**You rush yourself.**
You rely on urgency to overcome your slow operating speed. Over time this is exhausting.

# Workaround

**Anchor your attention in the present.**
Rushing usually involves anchoring attention in the future (vs. the present). Rushing toward the future may actually be more costly because you will have to make up for the *in-attentional* errors that occur when you are not in the present. Just a few minute minutes of meditation can help anchor you in the present. Practicing breathing techniques, taking breaks, and going outside are some other options.

*Anchor your attention in the present.*

# Obstacle

**You feel overwhelmed at the prospect of taking on a big task.**

# Workaround

**CHUNK IT!**
Break tasks into manageable segments and complete them one chunk at a time. This is the best strategy for making it easier to persist.

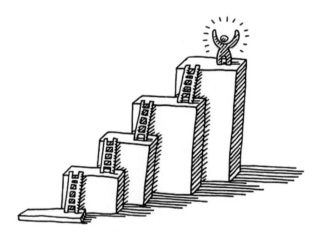

*Chunk It!*

# 10 Obstacle

**You expect success on the 1st try.**

# Workaround

**Your persistence is something you can control. Your performance, not so much.**

You have a performance disorder. Why put high expectations on your weakest link? The idea is to minimize weaknesses and maximize strengths. Your obstacle is that you are trying to do the opposite.

*Your persistence is something you can control.*
*Your performance, not so much.*

# By Illustration:

The author *allowed* himself to fail the psychologist exam 3 times (in order to pass the fourth time). I made a decision one day that I was going to pass the psychologist board exams. **My commitment was that I would keep taking these exams as many times as necessary until I passed.** This freed me from performance pressure. If I failed the exam I could retake it after a six-month wait, & there was no limit on how many times I could retake it.

The first time that I signed up to take the exam I had to have knee surgery a week before the exam. I decided that I would take the test anyway just for the experience. I studied for 2 days knowing, of course, that I would fail. It was such a wonderful experience walking into the examination room without any expectations. I had no anxiety. I couldn't fail as I knew that it was essentially impossible for me to pass. My score was indeed quite low, but not bad for someone who barely studied.

The second time I took the exam I studied for 2 weeks. (The recommended time to prepare for an exam like this was 3 to 6 months). I knew again that passing was a very low probability. I needed a score of 500 to pass and my score was 380. Not as bad as I thought it would be. The third time I took the exam I studied for one month. Again I knew that the odds of passing were still low. When the results came in I was just two points short of passing. After almost passing the third time, I knew that it was a possibility to pass it on the next try. This time I committed several months to prepare. When I drove to the exam center the forth time, the experience was very different than it had been the first time. I was listening to music rather than thinking about the test. I knew where to park. I knew where the bathroom was. I also knew that there was a good chance that I would pass the exam that day. But I also knew that if I didn't pass I would just take it again. I passed.

# Chapter 10 Summary
# Practicing Persistence

**DON'T GIVE UP!**

The more complicated the pathway toward a goal is, the <u>less</u> likely it is that that goal will actually be accomplished (if you have ADHD). Persistence can change this probability. Persistence, even at a very slow pace, is a powerful force. Think of glaciers. The successful adults in the resiliency study shared persistence as a common trait.

If you make sure you are on the right path toward a well-defined goal that you are motivated to accomplish, then the odds are that you will meet your goal if you don't give up.

Persistence is about not giving up in the face of obstacles. There are things within your control that you can do to enhance your ability to persist that don't involve suffering, deprivation or discipline. As a matter of fact, these things are more likely to involve fun, indulgence, and strategy.

The key to persistence is to make the journey sustainable over time. When you want to do something, it doesn't feel like work. Pathways that have fun built into them make it easier to persist. Breaking your goal into chunks can make it easier to persist. It is also important that you persist along pathways that actually lead you to your goal. There is no point in persisting on the road to nowhere!

It also helps to take the long view so as not to rush your self. Try to work at your own pace. Mainly, don't give up!

# Don't Give Up!

The author began working on this book 13 years before it was published.

# Integrative Summary of Book

## Taking control by working around ADHD, one obstacle at a time. A case example

This book is about taking control by working around ADHD, one obstacle at a time. I would like to sum up the book by telling you the story of Rachel, an amazing adult with ADHD who took control of her life. Since I don't want to compromise the identity of any real people that I have worked with, Rachel's story is actually an amalgamation of many actual stories. This is the account of how she took control of one aspect of her life by working around internal and external obstacles.

Rachel, 34, was diagnosed with ADHD later in life. Although she made many positive changes since being diagnosed, there was a particular area that still vexed her. It was something she had struggled with every month for years. Rachel was chronically late in paying her bills. She was paying huge late fees every month and her credit rating had been compromised.

Rachel's primary obstacle was her belief that her problem was laziness and a lack of discipline. Her plan involved becoming more disciplined in the future. Because she hadn't really factored in her ADHD, Rachel was tacitly setting herself up for failure. Her self-expectations were not aligned with her actual capacities, and she was erroneously trying to take control of her life by working around the wrong obstacles.

As a little girl Rachel was taught to view success as the byproduct hard work and discipline. She learned at an early age to rely on her rigid work ethic to make things happen. Unfortunately, hard work and discipline were not enough to prevent her from becoming swamped by the tsunami of challenges posed by inattention, restlessness and impulsivity. She would get caught up in the surge.

Then Rachel got help. She was motivated, and the changes that she made were extraordinary. Here is how she did it.

Rachel educated herself about ADHD. What she learned enabled her to reframe ADHD as a neurological disorder instead of a laziness disorder. She also learned that ADHD compromised her ability to estimate time accurately. She made the connection that bill paying involves the synchronization of performance and time. The more she learned the clearer it became that her struggle to remember to pay bills on time was related to ADHD, not a lack of discipline.

Rachel decided to monitor the process of bill paying so that she could craft workarounds based on what she observed. What she noticed first was her own judgment. She wasn't able to observe her bill-paying system without scolding herself, usually for not trying hard enough. Then she remembered reading that trying harder usually makes things worse if you have ADHD. That's when it hit her. "Of course, I had ADHD as a little girl too!" I always felt so bad about being *undisciplined*. "That poor little girl wasn't lazy or undisciplined," Rachel said to herself, "...she had ADHD." As Rachel began to take a closer, retrospective, look at her life it crystallized for her what it really means to be organizationally impaired. First she felt a sense of relief, and then came the sadness. It occurred to her that, in a way, she has been *trying hard* to *not have ADHD* her whole life instead of accepting herself the way she is and working around her limitations. She mourned the mountain of lost potentials and so many years trying to be somebody else. Rachel made big strides in terms of understanding, recognizing, and accepting her ADHD. She then made a vow to herself that she would learn to change this pattern by working around her ADHD in this area. Fortunately, she continued reading the chapters on goals, morale, and pathways to action. These chapters were exactly what she needed to revamp her ADHD-unfriendly bill paying system.

Rachel started by revisiting her goal. Her original goal had been to not to be late on her payments. Her goal of, *not being late* was a (less potent) negative goal, which needed revision. Rachel worked around this obstacle by constructing a more resonating, positive goal. Her new goal was to find a way to feel free and be financially responsible at the same time.

Rachel pictured herself in the future successfully working around her bill-paying obstacles. She imagined basking in the tranquility that comes with the knowledge that her bills had been paid (on time).

She decided that it would help to (literally) see her goal. She gathered some magazines and made a collage out of cutouts that represented her big-picture goal. She hung the collage in her bathroom as a visual reminder. The word *freedom* was written across the collage. It turned out that judgment was actually her main obstacle. Through her meditation practice Rachel began to pay attention to the extent of her self-judgment. It was pervasive. As she got better at labeling judgmental thoughts she noticed that she also felt calmer and safer. Calling judgment by its name seemed to reduce its power. Rachel decided that her morale and the quality of her life were more important than how she paid off her debt.

Rachel was now free to learn from trial and error since she got better at sidelining judgment. For the first time she was free to enjoy learning from her mistakes rather than avoid making them at all costs. She looked into some different pathways to action for paying bills online. One company was just too complicated and another was too expensive. The third was just right for Rachel. Of course there was a learning curve, but she eventually figured out how to transfer her bills to the bill-paying service. The end of the month arrived. No nasty voicemails. No drama. No problem. Rachel remembered her freedom collage. She remembered it because freedom is what she was feeling for the first time.

The new bill-paying system represented another *first* for Rachel in that she discovered a way to adapt the world to fit her needs rather than the other way around. She was always a round peg struggling to fit into a square hole. Trying to remember to pay the bills on time was bad for Rachel. Having a system where bills are paid automatically was a great fit for Rachel.

One of the interesting things about this story is the creative approach Rachel employed to accomplish the somewhat boring process of researching bill-paying services. Rachel paid her baby sitter to stay an extra two hours while she did her research. The baby sitter just sat in the same room and quietly did her homework, but her presence alone was enough to prompt Rachel to focus and get the job done amazingly quickly (45 minutes). It is hard to explain why this odd strategy worked. Rachel didn't care that this approach seemed mighty strange to every one she told it to. Well almost everyone.

One of the people she confided in was Bob, and he was not at all fazed by Rachel's baby-sitter strategy. As a matter of fact he said that he often hires high school students to come over when he has a boring job to do. "For some reason I always seem to get the job done whenever they come over," he said. Rachel had shivers down her spine. She was not used to resonating this much with someone without having to explain and/or defend herself. It turned out the Bob had ADHD too. She had never spoken frankly to another person with ADHD before. Soon she was talking to a number of strangely familiar people when Bob invited her to join his ADHD group. Rachel never felt more at home. Her warm connections to people like her provided her a foundation from which to build an ADHD-friendly future.

Rachel created the conditions that enabled her to persist until she achieved her goal. She didn't rush herself. She broke her tasks down into chunks. She was motivated to endure as she could see that she was truly on the right path to her goal. Hiring the baby sitter was a clever way to help her persist through some boring steps. Rachel had been persistent, but unfortunately she had persisted along the wrong path for many years (trying to become more disciplined). Now she persists on the right road, the road around her ADHD.

# References

Gerber, P.J. (2001). Employment of adults with learning disabilities and ADHD: Reasons for success and implications for resilience. The ADHD Report, 9, (4), pp 1-5. New York.

# Acknowledgments

What a delight it has been to work with fellow adults with ADHD. I have benefitted personally and professionally. Our collaborations have informed many of the ideas in this book. I would also like to thank my wife, Moon, both for her perpetual encouragement to keep writing this book, and for her valuable feedback once ideas were committed to the page. I would also like to express appreciation to Karrie Ross, my book designer, for patiently guiding me down the path toward actually getting this book published. Special thanks to Stephen Druker for his valuable editing and feedback.

# About the Author

Bill Rolfe Ph.D. is a licensed psychologist in private practice in West Los Angeles, California. He has been adjunct faculty at Phillips Graduate University for almost 30 years. For the past 12 years Dr. Rolfe has led specialized groups for high-functioning adults with ADHD. He has also led numerous workshops and seminars related working with adults with ADHD (including presentations at the international conferences for CHADD and ADDA).

www.DrBillRolfe.com

74839759R00071

Made in the USA
San Bernardino, CA
21 April 2018